300 Calorie or Less Light Meals

Quick and Easy '300 Calorie or Less' Meals

All Rights Reserved. No part of this publication may be reproduced in any form or by any means, including scanning, photocopying, or otherwise without prior written permission of the copyright holder. Copyright © 2014

Table of Contents

Introduction

Why 300-Calorie Recipes?

Foods to Avoid

300 Cal Light Meals

Chicken Soup
Emerald Soup
Quick Chicken Stir-Fry
Healthy Caesar Salad
Sweet Potato Shepherd's Pie
Cream of Broccoli Soup
Sweet and Sour Chicken
Asparagus with Prosciutto
Spicy Kale Quiche
Eggplant with Pesto Topping
Chilled Mango Soup
Mexican Tomato Soup
Spicy Mango Fried Rice

Kelp Noodle Salad

Zucchini Salad with Sundried Tomato Sauce

Spicy Tuna Tartare

Tilapia Ceviche

Spicy Kale with Poached Eggs

Smoked Salmon Bites

Basil Shrimp

Turkey Apple Wraps

Creamy Cauliflower Soup

Pineapple Jicama Salad

Sliced Veggie Spicy Chicken

No-Crust Pepper Quiche

Uptown Clam Chowder

Chicken & Kale Soup

Sweet Guava Salad

Carrot Cranberry Crunch Salad

300 Cal Snacks

Carrot Dip with Crudités

Sardine & Avocado on Endives

Sweet Potato Evening Bites

Chunked Apples

Black Pepper & Kale Chips

Tart Cherry Energy Bar

Simple Almond Apricot Balls

Bacon Wrapped Brussels Sprouts

Grilled Pineapple Fruit Salad

Spicy Chicken Bites

Coconut Shrimp

Green Goodness Smoothie

Mango Ginger Apple Salad

Avocado Banana Bread

Sweet Carrot Raisin Salad

Awesome Strawberry Salsa

Fresh Zesty Pico de Gallo

Fruit and Nut Apricot Pockets

Orange Cream Popsicles

Venison Teriyaki Skewers

Crunchy Eggplant Chips with Honey

Deer Jerky

Primal Cocoa Zucchini Muffin

Olive Tapenade

Gingerbread Cookies

Spicy Chicken Wraps

Tahini with Fruit Topping

Sugar Free Baked Apples

Ginger Mango Sherbet

Basic Banana Bread

Why 300-Calorie Recipes?

For some people, eating 3 square meals a day is not optimal for various reasons. To keep blood sugar stable, eating 6 smaller, 300-calorie meals per day is a popular option. By eating small meals, insulin spikes are kept under control, and blood sugar levels never drop because the body constantly receives food. This small-meal approach is used by many people who are physically active in order to sustain energy throughout the day. Some will prefer to have 3 small meals and a larger one, allowing for a greater variety of flavors and nutrients.

If you're looking at a 300-cal meal plan, there are a few things you need to know. Ideally, you will vary the foods from one meal to the other in order to get a wide array of nutrients. Eating 300 calories' worth of one food in one sitting, then eating 300 calories' worth of another food 2 hours later will likely cause you to miss out on vital nutrients found in a variety of foods. Creating simple yet nourishing 300-calorie meals is an art; balancing macronutrients (fat, protein and carbohydrates) along with micronutrients (vitamins, antioxidants and minerals) is the key to a successful 300-calorie meal.

Because some foods are very high in calories, they need to be avoided or consumed with moderation when aiming for 300-calorie meals. Nuts, avocado, oils, sugar, starches, grains, cheese and fatty meats such as bacon need to be limited because even a small amount of these foods will quickly burn through a 300-cal budget. The priority goes to chicken breast, eggs, lean fish, fruits, veggies and a little amount of fat. Soups, egg dishes and salads make excellent 300-calorie meals, but even stir-fries can be redesigned to fit the low-calorie guideline. Replacing the rice with grated cauliflower or swapping noodles for low-cal kelp noodles are creative ways to enjoy some waistline-friendly favorites.

The recipes in this book pack a ton of nutrition into a low-calorie package. You can enjoy each of them as part of a low-calorie wellness plan. If you wish, you can pair some of the soup options with a small spinach side salad drizzled with lemon juice or apple cider vinegar and a drop of olive oil for a complete low-calorie meal. Have fun experimenting with various combinations to create your own delicious and healthy meals!

Foods to Avoid

No food is off-limits, but you will generally want to avoid or limit:

- Pre-packaged foods: meal replacement bars, low-calorie frozen dinners and stuff that comes out of a can are not the best way to meet your daily nutrient needs. Loaded with sugar and preservatives, those foods leave you unsatisfied. Low-calorie prepared dinners are only low-cal because they come in tiny portions.
- Sugar: all sugar is high in calories and should be avoided. One tablespoon of honey adds 64 calories to your meal.
- Oils and fats: extra virgin oils such as olive and coconut oils can actually be consumed in moderation, even on a low-cal diet. While they are very high in calories, these fats contribute to good health in various ways. One tablespoon of oil contains upwards of 100 calories, so make sure you go easy. Avoid industrial and vegetable oils, avoid deep-fried anything, and save the oil for sautéing or as a salad garnish.
- Grains: grains have an obvious disadvantage when it comes to calories. They are made up of starches and sugars and their water content is relatively low, making them extremely high in calories. One cup of cooked pasta contains almost 200 calories, and not many people limit themselves to such a small amount. Likewise, 2 slices of wheat bread provide the same amount of calories, leaving very little room for extra nutrients.

300 Cal Light Meals

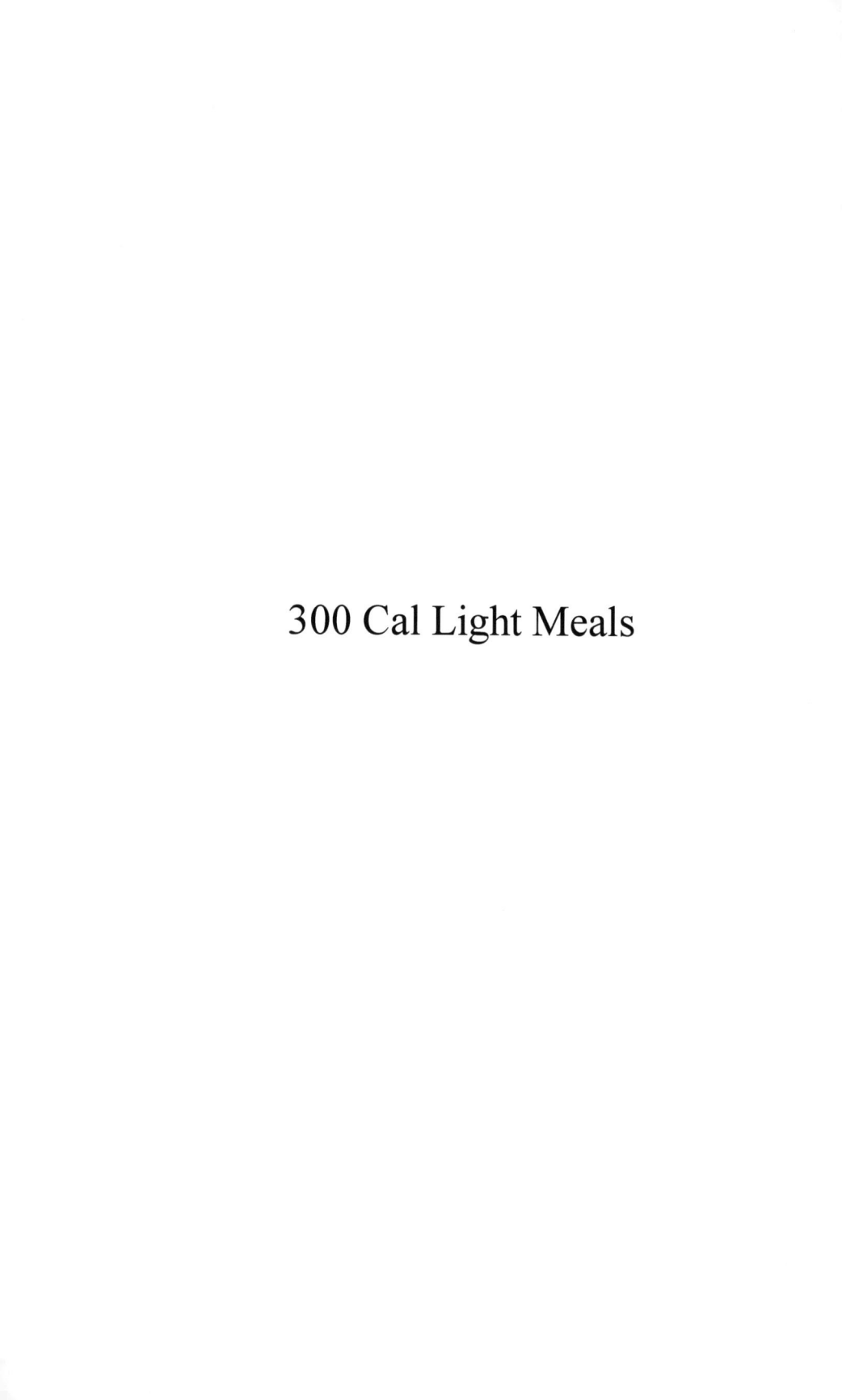

Creamy Parsnip Soup

Prep Time: 10 minutes

Cook Time: 25 minutes

Servings: 4

INGREDIENTS

1 large yellow onion, chopped

2 ripe pears, peeled and chopped

6 parsnips, peeled and chopped

4 cups chicken or vegetable broth

2 Tablespoons olive oil

1 teaspoon sea salt

INSTRUCTIONS

1. Sauté onion in olive oil in a large stockpot over medium-high heat until translucent.
2. Add parsnips, pears, broth, and salt.
3. Cover and bring to a boil.
4. Reduce heat to medium and simmer for approximately 20 minutes, until parsnips are tender.
5. Puree the soup with a hand blender, or in batches in a blender or food processor.

Chicken Soup

Prep Time: 10 minutes

Cook Time: 40 minutes

Servings: 4

INGREDIENTS

1 large yellow onion, chopped

4 garlic cloves, minced

2 carrots, chopped

2 stalks of celery, chopped

1 cup sliced mushrooms

½ cup parsley, chopped

4 cups chicken broth

2 skinless chicken legs

2 skinless chicken thighs

2 Tablespoons olive oil

1 teaspoon sea salt

INSTRUCTIONS

1. Sauté onion and garlic in olive oil in a large stockpot over medium heat until translucent.
2. Add the celery, carrots, and mushrooms and cook, stirring, for about 5 minutes.
3. Add the chicken legs and thighs, broth, parsley, and salt. Cover and simmer for 30 minutes.

Emerald Soup

Prep Time: 10 minutes
Cook Time: 25 minutes
Servings: 4

INGREDIENTS

2 large leeks, sliced
2 Tablespoons fresh ginger, grated
4 garlic cloves, minced
2 cups Chinese cabbage, chopped
4 cups fresh spinach
4 cups chicken or vegetable broth
2 Tablespoons coconut oil
1 teaspoon sea salt

INSTRUCTIONS

1. Sauté leeks in coconut oil in a large stockpot over medium-high heat about 5 minutes.
2. Add ginger and garlic, and stir, cooking, for another minute.
3. Add the cabbage, broth, and salt. Cover, and simmer for 20 minutes.
4. Add the spinach and stir in until wilted.

Quick Chicken Stir-Fry

Prep Time: 15 minutes
Cook Time: 20 minutes
Servings: 4

INGREDIENTS

1 pound chicken meat, cut into 1-inch chunks
1 yellow onion, sliced
2 carrots, peeled and sliced thinly
4 cups baby bok choy (about 2 heads), chopped
12 ounces mushrooms, halved
4 Tablespoons coconut oil
4 cloves garlic, chopped
1 Tablespoon grated ginger
1 Tablespoon apple cider vinegar.
1 teaspoon sea salt

INSTRUCTIONS

1. Sauté onions in coconut oil in a deep sauté pan or wok for about 3 minutes, or until translucent.
2. Add the chicken and cook, stirring frequently, until lightly browned.
3. Add the bok choy, carrots, and mushrooms and continue to sauté for a few minutes.
4. In a separate bowl, mix the vinegar, garlic, ginger, and salt, and whisk until blended.

5. Pour the sauce over the chicken and vegetables and cook, stirring frequently until vegetables are crisp-tender.

Potato-free Leek Soup

Prep Time: 15 minutes
Cook Time: 40 minutes
Servings: 4

INGREDIENTS

1 large yellow onion, chopped
2 large leeks, cleaned and sliced
1 large rutabaga, peeled and chopped
1 large head cauliflower, cored and chopped
6 cups chicken broth
2 Tablespoons olive oil
4 strips bacon (optional)
1 teaspoon sea salt

INSTRUCTIONS

1. Sauté onion in olive oil in a large stockpot over medium-high heat until translucent (about 4 minutes).
2. Add the leeks to the pot and cook, stirring, until lightly browned.
3. Add the rutabaga, cauliflower, salt, and stock to the pot. Bring to a boil.
4. Reduce heat to low, cover, and simmer for 30 minutes, until rutabaga is cooked through.
5. Puree the soup with a hand blender, or blender.

Healthy Caesar Salad

Prep Time: 5 minutes

Cook Time: 12 minutes

Servings: 2

INGREDIENTS

2 Tablespoons olive oil

2 Tablespoons lemon juice

4 anchovies

4 slices of bacon, diced

1 clove garlic, minced

4 cups romaine lettuce, torn

1 cup radicchio, torn

INSTRUCTIONS

1. Heat 1 Tablespoon oil in a skillet and sauté bacon until cooked, about 4-5 minutes.
2. In a blender or food processor, combine the remaining oil, the anchovies, and the lemon juice.
3. In a large bowl, toss the lettuce with the dressing and bacon.

Sweet Potato Shepherd's Pie

Prep Time: 10 minutes

Cook Time: 50 minutes

Servings: 4

INGREDIENTS

1 pound extra-lean ground turkey

1 large onion, chopped

2 medium zucchini, chopped

2 large sweet potatoes, peeled and diced

1 teaspoon dried thyme

1 teaspoon dried basil

2 Tablespoons olive oil

1 teaspoon sea salt

INSTRUCTIONS

1. Brown the meat with the onion in a large skillet. Cook until meat is fully cooked, about 15-20 minutes.
2. In another stockpot, steam sweet potatoes for about 20 minutes.
3. Add the zucchini and spices to the meat and cook for another 5 minutes.
4. Preheat oven to 400 °F.
5. Drain the sweet potatoes and return them to the pot. Mash with a potato masher and mix in the olive oil and sea salt.
6. Transfer the meat to a large casserole pan and pat it down with a spatula.

Sweet and Sour Chicken

Prep Time: 10 minutes

Cook Time: 20 minutes

Servings: 4

INGREDIENTS

1 pound skinless chicken breasts, cut into cubes

1 bunch scallions, chopped

1 cup pineapple, chopped (fresh or frozen)

2 large carrots, thinly sliced

2 stalks celery, sliced

½ pound mushrooms, halved

¼ cup apple cider vinegar

2 tablespoons coconut oil

1-inch piece of ginger, peeled and minced

2 cloves garlic, minced

INSTRUCTIONS
1. In a large skillet or walk, sauté the onions, celery, and garlic in the oil until soft, about 2 minutes.
2. Add the carrots, the mushrooms, the pineapple, and the chicken and continue stir-frying another 5 minutes.
3. Add the vinegar, cover, and reduce heat to low for 10 minutes.

Asparagus with Prosciutto

Prep Time: 10 minutes
Cook Time: 20 minutes
Servings: 4

INGREDIENTS

1 bunch asparagus, trimmed
2 Tablespoons plus 1 teaspoon olive oil
8 ounces prosciutto, thinly sliced
½ teaspoon sea salt

INSTRUCTIONS
1. Preheat oven to 400 °F.
2. Divide the asparagus spears into 8 bundles.
3. Wrap each bundle with 1/8 of the prosciutto and place on a baking sheet, lightly greased with 1 teaspoon olive oil.
4. Drizzle the remaining olive oil over the bundles and sprinkle with salt.
5. Bake for about 20 minutes, until asparagus is tender.

Spicy Kale Quiche

Prep time: 10 minutes

Cook time: 15 minutes

Serves: 4

INGREDIENTS

8 cage-free eggs

2 tbsp extra virgin olive oil

1 7oz bag of Kale greens

1 shallot

¼ tsp chipotle chili pepper powder

2 cloves garlic

½ lemon

2 tbsp coconut oil

¼ tbsp ground black pepper

INSTRUCTIONS

1. Place a steamer basket in the bottom of a large pot and fill with water; if you see water rise above the bottom of the basket, pour some out. Bring the water to a boil.
2. Wash the kale and remove the stems. Mince the garlic and shallot and squeeze the juice from the lemon into a bowl.

3. In a large pan, add the eggs and extra virgin olive oil. Mixing in the chipotle chili pepper powder, scramble the eggs, breaking them up until they form many small pieces, tender yet firm.
4. Place the kale in the pot and steam until tender and bright-green.
5. Remove the kale from the pot and combine with the eggs. Add the garlic, shallot and lemon juice, drizzle the coconut oil over top and add the ground black pepper. Mix and stir thoroughly.
6. Serve immediately or chill 20 minutes and then serve.

Eggplant with Pesto Topping

Prep time: 10 minutes

Cook time: 8 minutes

Serves: 4

INGREDIENTS

1 large, thick eggplant

6-8 tomatoes

4 tbsp olive oil

¼ cup fresh basil

2 cloves garlic

INSTRUCTIONS

1. Preheat the grill. Slice the eggplant lengthwise into ½" thick slices, or ensuring that you have 4 slices. Slice the tomatoes into ¼" thick slices. Combine 4 tbsp olive oil with basil and garlic in a food processor and puree together.
2. Grill the eggplant until browned, turning once, about 3-4 minutes per side.
3. Remove eggplant from the grill and lay the tomato slices out over each piece. Top with the pesto puree and serve.

Chilled Mango Soup

Prep Time: 10 minutes

Servings: 4

INGREDIENTS

3 large ripe mangoes

1 large onion (yellow, white or sweet)

2 inch piece fresh ginger

2 chili peppers

Cold water

INSTRUCTIONS

1. Peel mangoes, then carefully slice around pit. Peel and grate ginger. Peel and roughly chop onion. Remove stems and seeds from chilis, if desired.
2. Add to food processor or high-speed blender and process until smooth, about 2 minutes. Add enough water to reach desired consistency.
3. Transfer to serving dish and serve chilled.

Mexican Tomato Soup

Prep Time: 10 minutes

Cook Time: 40 minutes

Servings: 4

INGREDIENTS

2 cans (14.5 oz) organic crushed tomatoes

2 cans (11.5) organic tomato juice

5 large tomatoes (or 10 plum tomatoes)

1/2 cup chicken stock

1 red bell pepper (or 1/4 cup roasted red peppers, jarred)

1/4 red onion (or yellow or white onion)

2 garlic cloves

1/2 Serrano chili pepper (or other chili pepper) (optional)

1 tablespoon tapioca flour (or arrowroot powder)

2 tablespoons fresh Mexican oregano (or 1 teaspoon dried oregano)

2 large basil leaves

1 teaspoon fresh cracked black pepper (or ground black pepper)

Celtic sea salt, to taste

1 small bunch cilantro (for garnish)

2 tablespoons ghee (or bacon fat, cacao butter, or coconut oil)

INSTRUCTIONS

1. Juice tomatoes and set aside.

2. Roast red bell pepper over stove burner or until broiler, if using. Turn to char on all sides until skins sears. Rub off blackened skin. Cut in half and remove seeds, stem and veins.
3. Heat medium pot over medium-high heat. Add fat to hot pot.
4. Peel onion and garlic. Dice onion, roasted and red pepper. Mince garlic and Serrano pepper (optional). Add to hot oiled pot and sauté until fragrant, about 2 minutes.
5. Add tapioca and chicken stock. Stir to combine. Let cook about 2 minutes.
6. Chiffon (thinly slice) basil. Add to pot with tomato juice, crushed tomatoes, oregano, pepper and salt, to taste. Stir to combine.
7. Bring to simmer, then reduce heat to low. Simmer and reduce about 30 minutes, or until desired consistency is reached.
8. Transfer to serving dish. Chop cilantro and sprinkle over dish for garnish.
9. Serve hot.

Spicy Mango Fried Rice

Prep Time: 10 minutes

Cook Time: 15 minutes

Servings: 4

INGREDIENTS

1 head cauliflower

8 oz boneless, skinless chicken

1 mango

1 hot chili pepper

2 scallions

2 garlic cloves

3 tablespoons pure fish sauce (or coconut aminos)

3 teaspoons sesame oil (or walnut or almond oil)

1/2 teaspoon red pepper flake

1/2 lime

Coconut oil (for cooking)

INSTRUCTIONS

1. Heat large skillet or medium cast-iron wok over high heat. Lightly coat with coconut oil.
2. Cut cauliflower into florets and add to food processor with shredding attachment to rice. Or finely mince cauliflower.
3. Peel garlic and ginger and mince. Mince chili pepper. Thinly slice scallions. Carefully peel and dice mango. Dice chicken.

4. Add diced chicken, garlic, ginger, chili pepper and red pepper flake to hot skillet or wok. Sauté until chicken is golden brown and just cooked, about 3 minutes. Remove chicken and set aside.
5. Add cauliflower to hot pan or wok. Sauté about 5 minutes, until cauliflower is golden and a bit softened.

Kelp Noodle Salad

Prep Time: 5 minutes

Cook Time: 5 minutes

Servings: 2

INGREDIENTS

1 package (12 oz) kelp noodles

1/2 lemon

1 small cucumber

1 small red bell pepper

1 large carrot

Small bunch cilantro

2 large basil leaves

Orange Avocado Dressing

1 avocado

1 large orange

1/2 lemon

5 large basil leaves

1/4 teaspoon ground black pepper

1/4 teaspoon cayenne pepper or red pepper flake (optional)

Large bunch cilantro

INSTRUCTIONS

1. Rinse and drain kelp noodles. Add to medium bowl and soak 5 minutes in warm water and juice of 1/2 lemon. Or bring medium

pot of water with juice of 1/2 lemon to a boil and cook kelp noodles for 5 minutes, if softer texture preferred.
2. Peel, seed and cut cucumber in half width-wise. Cut bell pepper in half, then remove stem, seeds and veins. Use vegetable peeler or grater to make long, thin slices of carrot. Thinly slice cucumber and bell pepper lengthwise.
3. Add veggies and drained kelp noodles to medium mixing bowl.
4. For *Orange Avocado Dressing*, add basil and cilantro leaves to food processor or bullet blender with juice of orange and process to break down leaves. Slice avocado in half and remove pit. Scoop flesh into processor with juice of 1/2 lemon, black pepper and hot pepper (optional). Process until thick and until creamy.
5. Pour *Orange Avocado Dressing* over sliced veggies and kelp noodles. Toss to coat.
6. Serve immediately. Or refrigerate for 20 minutes and serve chilled.

Zucchini Salad with Sundried Tomato Sauce

Prep Time: 20 minutes*

Servings: 2

INGREDIENTS

1 medium zucchini

1 tomato

5 sundried tomatoes

1 garlic clove

2 fresh basil leaves

1 tablespoon raw virgin coconut oil (or 2 tablespoons warm water)

1/4 teaspoon ground white pepper (or black pepper)

1/4 teaspoon sea salt

INSTRUCTIONS

1. Run zucchini through spiralizer, slice into long, thin shreds with knife, or use vegetable peeler to make flat, thin slices. Sprinkle with a pinch of salt and pepper, and gently toss to coat.
2. Add tomato, sundried tomatoes, peeled garlic, basil, coconut oil or warm water, and remaining salt and pepper to food processor or bullet blender. Process until sauce of desired consistency forms.
3. Transfer zucchini pasta to serving bowls. Top with tomato sauce and serve immediately.
4. Or refrigerate for 20 minutes and serve chilled.

Spicy Tuna Tartare

Prep Time: 15* minutes

Servings: 4

INGREDIENTS

1 lb tuna steak (sushi grade)

1 small cucumber

1 ripe avocado

1 lime

1 garlic clove

1 hot chile pepper

2 tablespoons raw virgin coconut oil

Small bunch fresh cilantro

1 teaspoon red pepper flake

1 teaspoon sea salt

INSTRUCTIONS

1. Peel, seed and dice cucumber and avocado. Finely chop cilantro. Add to medium mixing bowl.
2. Remove seeds, stem and veins from hot pepper. Peel garlic and add to food processor or bullet blender with cayenne and hot pepper. Process until smooth paste forms. Add to bowl.
3. Dice tuna, discarding any tough white gristle. Add to bowl.
4. Squeeze on lime juice and add salt.
5. Gently toss with soft spatula or large spoon.
6. Serve immediately. Or refrigerate 20 minutes and serve chilled.

Tilapia Ceviche

Prep Time: 25 minutes

Servings: 4

INGREDIENTS

1 lb fresh, wild caught skinless tilapia fillets

Juice of 4 limes

Juice of 1 lemon

1 plum tomato

1/2 cucumber

1/2 small red onion

Medium bunch cilantro leaves

1/2 teaspoon sea salt

1/2 teaspoon ground black pepper

1 avocado

1 jalapeño pepper (optional)

INSTRUCTIONS

1. Dice fish with sharp knife. Freeze for 20 minutes to make cutting easier and cleaner, if preferred.
2. Add fish to medium mixing bowl. Juice all limes and 1/2 lemon over fish. Gently mix to combine. Cover and chill in refrigerator for 15 to 20 minutes, until fish is opaque.
3. Drain off liquid from fish and discard. Set fish aside.
4. Seed and dice tomato. Peel and dice cucumber and onion. Stem, seed and vein jalapeño pepper, then mince. Finely chop cilantro.

5. Add everything to marinated fish with salt and pepper. Juice remaining 1/2 lemon and mix to combine.
6. Slice avocado in half and pit and slice flesh.
7. Serve *Tilapia Ceviche* immediately with sliced avocado. Or refrigerate for 20 minutes and serve chilled.

Spicy Kale with Poached Eggs

Prep time: 10 minutes

Cook time: 12 minutes

INGREDIENTS

1 handful kale

2 cage-free eggs

1 small onion

1 clove garlic

1 tbsp extra virgin olive oil

¼ tsp ground black pepper

1 tsp low-sodium horseradish (optional)

INSTRUCTIONS

1. Chop the onion and mince the garlic. De-stem and wash the kale. Leaving a bit of water on the kale is ideal.
2. In a saucepan, add 1 tbsp extra virgin olive oil over medium heat. Add onion and cook until it begins to lose its opaqueness, about 5 minutes.
3. Add kale to saucepan and cover until kale is soft and green, about 5 minutes. Add garlic and stir, then cook another 2 minutes and remove from heat.
4. Fill a saucepan half full of water. Bring the water to a boil, then reduce heat below a boil and hold it there.
5. One by one, crack the eggs into a small cup or bowl and, with the lip of the cup or bowl close to the water's surface, dump the egg

into the water. If necessary, nudge the eggwhites closer to the yolks to keep them together.
6. Once all the eggs are in the water, remove the pan from heat and cover it. Let sit for 4 minutes until all eggs are cooked, then remove eggs from pan.
7. Place the greens on a plate and the two eggs on top of the greens. Top with horseradish if desired. Serve.

Smoked Salmon Bites

Prep Time: 10 minutes

Cook Time: N/A

Servings: 2

INGREDIENTS

1 large seedless cucumber

4 oz smoked salmon

1 avocado

½ red onion

1 Tablespoon lemon juice

1/2 teaspoon sea salt

Chives for garnish (optional)

INSTRUCTIONS

1. Slice the cucumber into ¾-inch thick slices.
2. Slice the smoked salmon into 1-inch by 1-inch pieces.
3. In a small bowl, mash the avocado with the salt, lemon juice, and onion.
4. Spread the avocado mash evenly across each of the cucumber slices.
5. Top each cucumber with a piece of the smoked salmon.
6. Garnish with a chive, if desired.

Basil Shrimp

Prep Time: 5 minutes

Cook Time: 20 minutes

Servings: 4

INGREDIENTS

1 pound shrimp, cleaned, tails on

1 Tablespoon coconut oil

1 bunch green onions, trimmed and chopped

1 cup fresh basil leaves

2 cloves garlic, sliced

2 Tablespoons lime juice

INSTRUCTIONS

1. In a large skillet, sauté the onions and garlic 2-3 minutes.
2. Add the shrimp and stir-fry for another 3-5 minutes, until cooked through.
3. Add the basil and lime juice and simmer another 2-3 minutes.

Turkey Apple Wraps

Prep Time: 5 minutes

Cook Time: N/A

Servings: 2

INGREDIENTS

8 ounces nitrite-free turkey lunch meat

1 apple, sliced into 8 spears

1 avocado, sliced into 8 pieces lengthwise

1 cup watercress

INSTRUCTIONS

1. Divide the turkey into fourths.
2. Lay one-fourth of the watercress, apple, and avocado lengthwise in the center of each piece of meat.
3. Roll up tightly and serve whole or slice each roll into bite-sized pieces.

Creamy Cauliflower Soup

Prep Time: 10 minutes
Cook Time: 20 minutes
Servings: 4

INGREDIENTS

1 large white onion, chopped
4 cloves garlic, minced
1 large head cauliflower, cored and chopped
4 cups chicken or vegetable stock
2 Tablespoons olive oil
4 strips bacon (optional)
1 teaspoon sea salt

INSTRUCTIONS

1. Sauté onion in olive oil in a large stockpot over medium-high heat until translucent (about 4 minutes).
2. Add the cauliflower, garlic, salt, and stock to the pot. Bring to a boil.
3. Reduce heat to low, cover, and simmer for 8-10 minutes.
4. While soup is simmering, pan fry the bacon strips (if using) until crispy.
5. Puree the soup with a hand blender, or blender.
6. Serve in bowls, crumbling the bacon on top.

Pineapple Jicama Salad

Prep Time: 5 minutes

Cook Time: N/A

Servings: 4

INGREDIENTS

1 small red onion, thinly sliced

2 cups jicama, peeled and diced

2 cups pineapple, peeled, cored, and chopped

4 cups red cabbage, shredded

2 Tablespoons lime juice

2 Tablespoons olive oil

½ cup fresh mint leaves

1 teaspoon sea salt

INSTRUCTIONS

1. In a bowl, combine the onion, jicama, pineapple, and mint.
2. In a separate bowl, whisk the olive oil, lime juice, and salt.
3. Serve the salad on a bed of red cabbage and drizzle the dressing over it before serving.

Sliced Veggie Spicy Chicken

Prep time: 4 minutes

Cook time: 8 minutes

Servings: 4

INGREDIENTS

4 pieces skinless grass-fed chicken thighs

1 onion

2 cloves garlic

3/4 cup sliced carrots

2 handfuls Kale greens

2 tbsp chinese five spice

2 tbsp smoked paprika

2 tbsp chipotle chili pepper powder

1 tbsp olive oil

2 tsp lemon juice

1 tbsp coconut oil

INSTRUCTIONS

1. Mince garlic and chop onion to desired size (medium strips work best). Chop carrots to 1/4" thickness. De-rib the kale and chop it coarsely, wash it and allow water to remain on the leaves. Bring 4 cups of water to a light boil.
2. Heat 1 tbsp olive oil over medium heat in a large pan. Add carrot and onion and cook for 8 minutes, stirring occasionally.

3. Meanwhile, heat 1 tbsp coconut oil over medium heat in a separate pan. Add chicken and cook for 4 minutes. Season chicken with chinese five spice, chipotle chili pepper powder and smoked paprika and turn, adding more of each spice to the other side of the chicken, cooking for another 4 minutes or until cooked through.
4. Add kale to boiling water and boil until bright green, about 5 minutes. Remove from water and let sit while the vegetables and chicken continue cooking.
5. Add everything into the pan with the vegetables and add 2 tsp lemon juice. Add minced garlic and stir for 1 minute.
6. Serve immediately.

No-Crust Pepper Quiche

Prep time: 5 minutes

Cook time: 3-6 minutes

INGREDIENTS

2 cage-free eggs

1 small onion

1 clove garlic

½ red bell pepper

1 tbsp extra virgin olive oil

¼ tsp smoked paprika

¼ tsp ground black pepper

INSTRUCTIONS

1. Finely chop onion, garlic and red bell pepper.
2. Pour extra virgin olive oil into a pan over medium heat.
3. Crack eggs and pour into a small bowl. Combine with onion, garlic and red bell pepper and whisk until mixed together.
4. Pour contents of bowl into pan and add smoked paprika and ground black pepper. Scramble until desired doneness.
5. Serve.

Uptown Clam Chowder

Prep Time: 10 minutes

Cook Time: 1 hour 15 minutes

Servings: 4

INGREDIENTS

24 - 36 medium live littleneck clams (or other clam varieties)

2 cans (11.5) organic tomato juice (or about 6 large tomatoes)

2 cans (14.5 oz) organic crushed tomatoes

2 medium carrots

2 medium celery stalks

2 medium parsnips

1 red bell pepper

1 tablespoon tamari (or coconut aminos or liquid aminos)

1 bay leaf

1/4 teaspoon cayenne pepper

1/2 teaspoon onion powder

1 tablespoon dried oregano

1 tablespoon dried basil

1 teaspoon dried thyme

1 teaspoon ground black pepper

Celtic sea salt, to taste

1 cup clam juice (or veggie or chicken stock, or water) (optional)

INSTRUCTIONS

1. Have fishmonger shuck clams. Or carefully shuck clams yourself. Reserve clam juice. Set aside in refrigerator.
2. Juice tomatoes, if using. Add tomato juice and crushed tomatoes to medium pot. Heat pot over high heat.
3. Remove seeds, stems and veins from bell pepper. Dice bell pepper, carrot, celery, and parsnips. Add to pot with spices and salt, to taste.
4. Bring pot to boil, then reduce heat to low. Place lid loosely over pot to prevent splatter. Simmer for 45 minutes. Stir occasionally.
5. Remove lid and stir. Add clam juice, stock or water to reach desired consistency (optional).
6. Remove clams from refrigerator and chop, if desired. Add clams and juice to pot. Stir to combine.
7. Replace lid and continue cooking about 20 - 30 minutes. Stir occasionally.
8. Transfer to serving dish and serve hot.

Chicken & Kale Soup

Prep Time: 10 minutes

Cook Time: 35 minutes

Servings: 4

INGREDIENTS

1 pound chicken breasts, cooked and shredded

6 cups chicken broth

1 large bunch kale, chopped

2 parsnips, peeled and diced

1 yellow onion, chopped

2 cloves garlic, sliced

2 Tablespoons olive oil

1 lemon, juiced

INSTRUCTIONS

1. Sauté onion in a large stockpot over medium-high heat in the olive oil until translucent, about 5 minutes.
2. Add the chicken, broth, kale, garlic, and parsnips. Bring to a boil. Lower heat, and simmer 20-30 minutes
3. Add the lemon juice just before serving

Sweet Guava Salad

Prep Time: 10 minutes*

Servings: 2

INGREDIENTS

2 ripe guavas

1 personal papaya (1 cup diced papaya flesh)

1 young coconut

1/2 teaspoon ground ginger (or 1/4 inch piece fresh ginger)

2 tablespoons fresh orange juice (about 1/2 orange)

INSTRUCTIONS

1. Dice guavas and add to medium mixing bowl. Peel papaya and cut in half, remove seeds and dice flesh. Remove coconut flesh from shell and dice. Add to bowl.
2. Juice orange into bowl and add ground ginger. Or peel fresh ginger and mince, then add to bowl. Toss to coat fruit evenly.
3. Transfer to serving dishes and serve immediately.
4. *Or refrigerate for 20 minutes and serve chilled.

Carrot Cranberry Crunch Salad

Prep Time: 5 minutes

Servings: 1

INSTRUCTIONS

2 large carrots

3 tablespoon dried cranberries

3 tablespoons raw almonds

1/2 small orange (or tangerine)

1/2 piece fresh ginger

1/2 teaspoon ground ginger

DIRECTIONS

1. Add carrots to food processor with shredding attachment and process, or grate with grater. Add to medium mixing bowl with cranberries and ground ginger.
2. Add almonds to food processor and pulse to coarsely chop. Or add to paper or plastic kitchen bag and pound with heavy rolling pin to crush. Peel ginger and dice or finely grate. Zest *then* juice orange. Add to carrot mixture and toss to combine.
3. Transfer to serving dish and serve immediately. Or refrigerate 20 minutes and serve chilled.

300 Cal Snacks

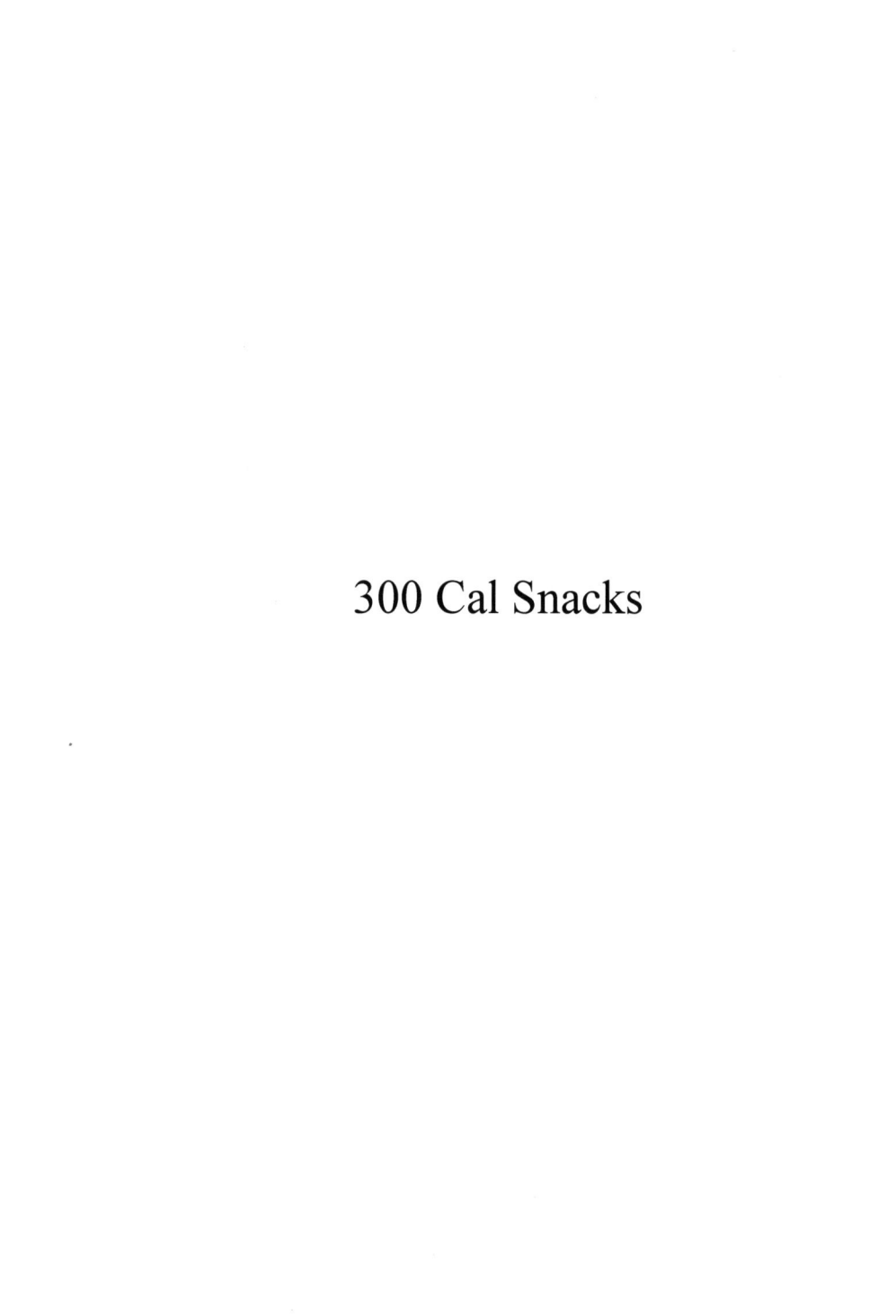

Carrot Dip with Crudités

Prep Time: 10 minutes

Cook Time: 10 minutes

Servings: 4

INGREDIENTS

1 pound carrots, cut into 1-inch chunks

2 Tablespoons coconut oil

1 clove garlic, minced

1 teaspoon ginger, minced

½ teaspoon sea salt

1 Tablespoon lemon juice

Crudités for serving: Broccoli or Cauliflower florets, Sliced Jicama, Asparagus, Green beans, Cucumber spears, etc.

INSTRUCTIONS

1. Bring a small pot of water to a boil and boil the carrots 8-10 minutes, until soft. Drain and rinse.
2. Add all of the dip ingredients to a blender or food processor and pulse to combine.
3. Serve the dip with a variety of crudités for dipping.

Sardine & Avocado on Endives

Prep Time: 5 minutes
Cook Time:
Servings: 4

INGREDIENTS

1-2 bunches endives
1 tin sardines in olive oil
1 Tablespoon apple cider vinegar
1 Tablespoon lemon juice
2 Tablespoons fresh parsley
1 avocado, halved, pitted, and chopped
½ teaspoon sea salt

INSTRUCTIONS

1. In a medium bowl, combine the sardines, vinegar, parsley, and lemon juice. Marinate the sardines for about 30 minutes in the refrigerator.
2. In the meantime, remove the leaves from the endives, wash them, and pat them dry. Set them on a platter, with the "cup" side facing up.
3. After the sardines are chilled, mix in the avocados. Use a spoon to divide the mixture among the endive leaves. There should be enough mixture to fill about 12 leaves.

Sweet Potato Evening Bites

Prep time: 10 minutes

Cook time: 30 minutes

INGREDIENTS

3 sweet potatoes

¼ cup extra virgin olive oil

¼ tsp Celtic sea salt

¼ tsp smoked paprika

INSTRUCTIONS

1. Preheat oven to 500 degrees.
2. Peel the potatoes and cut them into small wedges. In a large bowl, combine potato wedges, extra virgin olive oil, Celtic sea salt and smoked paprika. Mix well until all wedges are coated in all ingredients.
3. Place on a baking sheet and bake for 30 minutes, turning once halfway through, and continue cooking until they are well browned.
4. Remove from oven and let cool. Serve.

Chunked Apples

Prep time: 10 minutes

Cook time: 10-15 minutes

INGREDIENTS

1 cup grapes

1 tsp arrowroot

½ cup water

3 large apples

INSTRUCTIONS
1. Boil water in a small saucepan.
2. Add the grapes to the water and boil until soft, about 2-3 minutes.
3. Cool the mixture; blend it and then strain, removing excess water.
4. In a pan, combine arrowroot, ½ cup water, and grape mixture.
5. Simmer until the mixture turns slightly thick and remove from heat.
6. Slice the apples in half and hollow out a decent portion surrounding the core.
7. Place an equal amount of grape mixture into the hollowed portion of each apple chunk.
8. Serve.

Black Pepper & Kale Chips

Prep time: 15 minutes

Cook time: 10-15 minutes

INGREDIENTS

1 handful baby kale greens

¼ tsp garlic powder

2 tbsp coconut oil

¼ tsp Celtic sea salt

¼ tsp ground black pepper

INSTRUCTIONS

1. Preheat oven to 350 degrees.
2. In a large bowl, combine 2 tbsp melted coconut oil with kale greens, garlic powder, Celtic sea salt and ground black pepper. Mix well.
3. Line a baking sheet with parchment paper and place kale on it. Bake until the edges of the kale are browned, 10-15 minutes.
4. Remove from oven and cool. Serve.

Tart Cherry Energy Bar

Prep Time: 25 minutes

Servings: 6

INGREDIENTS

1 cup dried tart cherries

1/4 cup dried pitted dates

1/3 cup warm water

1 lime

1 cup raw almonds

1/4 teaspoon ground ginger

1/4 teaspoon vanilla

1/8 teaspoon Celtic sea salt

INSTRUCTIONS

1. Zest and juice lime into small mixing bowl. Add warm water and dried cherries. Toss to coat and set aside 10 minutes.
2. Line loaf pan with parchment paper.
3. Add nuts and dates to food processor or high-speed blender. Drain soaked cherries and add to processor with cinnamon, vanilla and salt. Process for about 1 minute, until mixture is coarsely ground and sticks together when pressed.
4. Scrape mixture into prepared loaf pan and press firmly into bottom with hands or spatula.
5. Place in refrigerator and chill for 10 minutes. Remove and cut into 6 bars.

6. Serve immediately. Or store in refrigerator up to 2 weeks.

Simple Almond Apricot Balls

Prep Time: 15 minutes

Servings: 12

INGREDIENTS

1/2 cup dried pitted dates

1/3 cup dried apricots

1/3 cup almonds (toasted or roasted, if preferred)

1/4 cup flaked or shredded coconut

1/2 tablespoon raw honey (or agave)

INSTRUCTIONS

1. Add apricots and dates to food processor or high-speed blender. Process until finely chopped, about 1 - 2 minutes.
2. Add almonds and coconut to processor. Process until well ground, about 2 minutes. Add honey and pulse until mixture sticks together, about 30 seconds.
3. Form mixture into 12 balls.
4. Serve immediately. Or store in airtight container in refrigerator up to 2 weeks.

Bacon Wrapped Brussels Sprouts

Prep Time: 10 minutes

Cook Time: 20 minutes

Servings: 4

INGREDIENTS

24 Brussels sprouts

8 strips nitrate-free bacon

24 wooden toothpicks

1/4 teaspoon ground black pepper

INSTRUCTIONS

1. Preheat oven to 375 degrees F. Place oven-safe wire rack in sheet pan.
2. Soak toothpicks in water for about 5 minutes.
3. Cut bacon strips into thirds. Wrap each Brussels sprout in bacon and use toothpicks to secure.
4. Place bacon wrapped Brussels sprouts on wire rack and sprinkle with pepper.
5. Bake for about 15 - 20 minutes, until bacon is crisp and veggies are cooked through. Remove and let cool about 2 minutes.
6. Serve warm or room temperature.

Grilled Pineapple Fruit Salad

Prep Time: 5 minutes
Cook Time: 10 minutes
Servings: 4

INGREDIENTS

1/2 pineapple
1 peach
1 cup fresh cherries
1 orange
1 tablespoon fresh mint leaves
Half lemon

INSTRUCTIONS

1. Heat griddle or grill over medium-high heat. Lightly coat with coconut oil.
2. Peel and core pineapple. Cut into half inch slices. Place slice on griddle and grill about 4 - 5 minutes on each side, until grill marks appear and sugars caramelized.
3. Cut peach in half and grill flesh side down for about 5 minutes.
4. Pit cherries and slice in half. Peel orange and cut flesh from white cellulose film and pith.
5. Chop pineapple and peach. Add to medium mixing bowl with cherries and orange wedges. Chiffon mint. Add to bowl and squeeze on lemon juice. Toss to combine.
6. Serve room temperature. Or refrigerate and serve chilled.

Spicy Chicken Bites

Prep Time: 5 minutes

Cook Time: 10 minutes

Servings: 4

INGREDIENTS

8 oz boneless skinless chicken

1/2 cup almond meal

1 teaspoon flax meal

1 teaspoon paprika

1/2 teaspoon cayenne pepper

1/2 teaspoon red pepper flakes

1/2 teaspoon ground black pepper

1/2 teaspoon sea salt

1 egg

1 jalapeño pepper

2 garlic cloves

2 oz organic spicy brown mustard

Coconut oil (for cooking)

INSTRUCTIONS

1. Heat a medium skillet over medium high heat. Lightly coat pan with coconut oil.
2. Slice chicken into 1x1 inch strips. Arrange slices between 2 sheets of parchment and pound with kitchen mallet or rolling pin to

flatten slightly. Place flattened pieces between two paper towels to absorb excess moisture.
3. In a shallow dish, blend almond meal, flax meal, dry spices and salt.
4. Add egg, jalapeño and peeled garlic to food processor or bullet blender. Process until fairly smooth. Pour into shallow dish.
5. Dip chicken pieces into jalapeño egg, then dredge in seasoned almond meal.
6. Carefully place coated chicken pieces into hot oil and fry about 2 minutes, until golden brown and cooked through. Turn with tongs half way through.
7. Drain cooked chicken on paper towel, then transfer to serving dish.
8. Serve hot with spicy mustard.

Coconut Shrimp

Prep Time: 10 minutes
Cook Time: 15 minutes
Servings: 4

INGREDIENTS

3 egg whites

1 lb large shrimp

1 cup flaked coconut

1/2 teaspoon garlic powder

1/2 teaspoon ground white pepper (or ground black pepper)

1 teaspoon sea salt

Coconut oil (for cooking)

Mango Salsa

1 ripe mango

1/2 small white onion

1 small jalapeño

Juice of half lime

INSTRUCTIONS

1. Preheat oven to 425 degrees F. Line sheet pan with parchment paper. Or place oven-safe wire rack over sheet pan.
2. Add coconut to shallow dish.
3. Beat egg whites with salt, pepper and garlic powder in a large mixing bowl with hand mixer or whisk until light and fluffy.

4. Peel and devein shrimp. Leave tails on. Add shrimp to egg whites to coat.
5. Let excess egg white drain from shrimp, then add to coconut flakes. Toss to coat. Return shrimp to egg whites, then coconut flakes again. Press shrimp into coconut and coat well.
6. Place the shrimp on prepared sheet pan. Brush lightly with liquid coconut oil.
7. Place in oven and bake for 5 - 7 minutes. Then turn shrimp over, brush with coconut oil, and bake another 5 - 7 minutes, until coconut is golden brown and shrimp are bright pink.
8. For *Mango Salsa*, slice mango around pit. Peel and dice flesh. Peel and dice onion. Mince jalapeño, discarding seeds and stem. Add to small serving dish juice of half a lime. Mix to combine.
9. Remove shrimp from oven and allow to cool for a few minutes.
10. Serve warm with *Mango Salsa*.

Green Goodness Smoothie

Prep Time: 5 minutes

Servings: 2

INGREDIENTS

2 cups spinach

2 whole kale leaves (1 cup chopped)

1 banana

1 green apple

1/2 cup green grapes

1 cup water (or fresh nut milk)

INSTRUCTIONS

1. Remove stems and ribs from kale. Core apple and dice. Peel banana.
2. Add water, banana and grapes to full sized blender. Process until solids are broken down.
3. Add greens and pulse on low for 30 seconds to break down. Then process on high for 1 minute, until smooth.
4. Pour into serving glasses and serve immediately.
5. Or chill in refrigerator for 20 minutes, blend for a few seconds to incorporate separated liquid, then pour into serving glasses and serve chilled.

Mango Ginger Apple Salad

Prep Time: 5 minutes

Servings: 2

INSTRUCTIONS

1 ripe mango

1 granny smith apple

1/4 cup raw cashews

1 inch piece fresh ginger

1/2 teaspoon ground ginger

INGREDIENTS

1. Slice mango in half around pit. Peel flesh and dice. Add to small mixing bowl.
2. Core apple and dice. Peel ginger and mince. Add to bowl with ground ginger.
3. Roughly chop cashews and add to bowl.
4. Mix well and serve immediately. Or refrigerate 20 minutes and serve chilled.

Avocado Banana Bread

Prep Time: 5 minutes

Cook Time: 25 minutes

Servings: 9

INGREDIENTS

3/4 cup almond flour

1/4 cup coconut flour

2 tablespoons flax meal (or ground chia seed)

2 eggs

1 large overripe banana

1 avocado

1/4 cup sweetener*

2 tablespoons coconut oil

1 tablespoon baking powder

1 tablespoon cinnamon

1 teaspoon ground ginger

1 teaspoon vanilla

1/2 teaspoon ground black pepper

1/2 teaspoon sea salt

1/2 cup organic banana chips (optional)

INSTRUCTIONS

1. Preheat oven to 350 degrees F. Coat square baking pan with coconut oil.

2. Slice avocado in half. Remove pit and scoop flesh into medium mixing bowl. Peel banana and add to bowl with eggs, sweetener, and flax or chia meal. Beat with hand mixer or whisk until well blended.
3. Sift flour, baking powder, salt and spices Into banana mixture. Mix until combined. Roughly chop banana chips and fold into batter (optional).
4. Pour batter into baking pan and bake for 20 - 25 minutes, or until browned and firm in the center.
5. Remove from oven and let cool at least 5 minutes.
6. Slice and serve warm. Or allow to cool completely and serve room temperature.

NOTE: Bake in oiled loaf pan for 35 - 45 minutes for **Avocado Banana Loaf**.

stevia, raw honey or agave nectar

Sweet Carrot Raisin Salad

Prep Time: 5 minutes
Servings: 2

INSTRUCTIONS

2 large carrots
2 tablespoons red raisins
2 tablespoons golden raisins
1/4 cup raw slivered almonds (or sliced almonds)
1/2 small orange (or tangerine)
1/4 teaspoon ground cinnamon

DIRECTIONS

1. Add carrots to food processor with shredding attachment and process, or grate with grater. Add to medium mixing bowl with raisins, almonds and cinnamon.
2. Zest *then* juice orange. Add to carrot mixture and toss to combine.
3. Transfer to serving dishes and serve immediately. Or refrigerate 20 minutes and serve chilled.

Awesome Strawberry Salsa

Prep Time: 5 minutes*

Servings: 4

INGREDIENTS

2 cups fresh strawberries

1/2 small white onion

1/4 red bell pepper

Medium bunch fresh mint

1/2 lime

1/2 orange

1/2 teaspoon ground black pepper

INSTRUCTIONS

1. Remove strawberry stems and leaves, then finely dice. Add to medium mixing bowl.
2. Peel onion and finely dice. Remove mint leave s from stem then chiffon, or thinly slice. Add to strawberries with pepper and squeeze of lime and orange. Mix until well combined.
3. Transfer mixture to serving dish and serve immediately with raw chips. Or refrigerate for 20 minutes and serve chilled.

Fresh Zesty Pico de Gallo

Prep Time: 15 minutes*

Servings: 4

INGREDIENTS

4 plum tomatoes

1/2 small red onion

Small bunch fresh cilantro

1/2 jalapeño pepper

1/2 lime

1 garlic clove

1/8 teaspoon garlic powder

1/4 teaspoon ground cumin

1/4 teaspoon Celtic sea salt

1/4 teaspoon ground black pepper

INSTRUCTIONS

1. Finely dice tomatoes. Peel and dice onion. Add to medium mixing bowl.
2. Finely chop cilantro. Remove seeds, veins and stem from jalapeño, then mince. Peel and mince garlic. Add to tomatoes with salt, spices and squeeze of lime. Mix until well combined.
3. Transfer mixture to serving dish
4. *Refrigerate 3 hours. Serve room temperature or chilled with raw chips.

Fruit and Nut Apricot Pockets

Prep Time: 10 minutes

Servings: 4

INGREDIENTS

1 cup dried apricots

1/4 cup raw cashews

2 - 3 tablespoons dried cranberries

2 - 3 tablespoons dried blueberries

INSTRUCTIONS

1. Roughly chop cashews and add too small mixing bowl with cranberries and blueberries. Mix to combine.
2. Open apricots slightly to reveal pocket. Take pinch of mixed nuts and fruit and stuff apricots. Leave a little room to pinch apricot closed.
3. Transfer to serving dish and serve immediately. Or store in airtight container.

Orange Cream Popsicles

Prep Time: 10 minutes*

Servings: 12

INGREDIENTS

2 cups orange or tangerine juice (about 9 oranges or 15 tangerines)

1/2 cup shredded or flaked coconut (or 1 mature coconut)

Water

Ice pop maker, toothpicks or popsicle sticks

INSTRUCTIONS

1. *Freeze ice pop maker or ice cube tray for at least 30 minutes.
2. *Soak flaked coconut in 2/3 - 3/4 cups water at least 6 hours, or overnight in refrigerator.
3. Add soaked coconut and soaking liquid to food processor or high-speed blender.
4. Or remove flesh from fresh coconut and add to high-speed blender with 2/3 - 3/4 cups water. Process until well blended and fairly smooth, about 1 - 2 minutes.
5. Strain mixture through nut milk bag, cheesecloth or strainer back into blender. Reserve pulp and set aside to dry and dehydrate, then use as coconut flour.
6. Juice oranges and add to blender. Process until well combined, about 30 seconds.
7. Remove ice pop maker or ice cube tray from freezer. Pour mixture into wells and fill 3/4 full. Place in freezer about 20 minutes.

8. Place ice pop maker sticks, toothpicks or popsicle sticks into well. Return to freezer about 20 minutes.
9. Remove ice pops from freezer and serve immediately.

Venison Teriyaki Skewers

Prep Time: 10 minutes*
Cook Time: 10 minutes
Servings: 4

INGREDIENTS

16 oz (1 lb) venison

1 bell pepper

1 cup pearl onions

12 wooden skewers (soaked in water for 1 hour)

Teriyaki Marinade

1/4 cup pure fish sauce (or tamari or coconut aminos)

2 tablespoons apple cider vinegar (or liquid aminos or coconut vinegar)

2 tablespoons raw honey (or agave)

1 tablespoon sesame oil (or coconut, walnut or almond oil)

2 garlic cloves

1 inch piece fresh ginger root

1/4 teaspoon red pepper flakes (optional)

Coconut oil (for cooking)

INSTRUCTIONS

1. Cut venison into 1 inch chunks. Remove stems, seeds and veins from bell pepper, then roughly chop. Peel pearl onions.

2. For *Teriyaki Marinade*, peel and mince garlic and ginger. Add to medium mixing bowl with fish sauce, vinegar, honey, sesame oil and red pepper (optional).
3. *Add venison, peppers and onions to *Teriyaki Marinade* and toss to coat. Cover and set aside to marinate for 1 hour.
4. *Soak wooden skewers in water in shallow dish for 1 hour.
5. Preheat outdoor grill or griddle pan over medium-high heat. Lightly coat with coconut oil.
6. Drain marinade from meat and veggies. Pierce venison, peppers and onions with soaked skewers, alternating meat and veggies.
7. Cook skewers on preheated grill about 1 - 2 minutes per side, for medium well. Turn several times while cooking. Do not overcook.
8. Remove skewers from heat and transfer to serving dish.
9. Serve hot.

Crunchy Eggplant Chips with Honey

Prep Time: 10 minutes

Cook Time: 20 minutes

Servings: 4

INGREDIENTS

1 medium eggplant

2 cage-free eggs

1/3 cup almond flour (or almond meal)

1/3 cup coconut flour

1/4 cup arrowroot powder

1 teaspoon ground black pepper

1 teaspoon Celtic sea salt

1/4 cup raw honey (or agave)

Coconut oil (for cooking)

Water

INSTRUCTIONS

1. Heat medium pan over medium-high heat. Coat pan with 1/4 inch coconut oil.
2. Cut off ends of eggplant. Carefully slice eggplant crosswise into thin slices about 1/8 inch thick with sharp knife or mandolin. Sprinkle with 1/2 teaspoon salt and pepper.
3. Add arrowroot powder to shallow dish. In separate shallow dish, blend almond flour, coconut flour and remaining salt and pepper. Whisk eggs in small mixing bowl or third shallow dish.

4. Dredge eggplant slices in arrowroot, shaking off excess. Dip dusted eggplant into egg, turning several times to coat. Shake off excess and dredge eggplant in flour mixture and coat well. Transfer to large dish for storage between steps.
5. Carefully place coated eggplant in hot oil and cook 1 - 2 minutes on each side, until golden brown and crisp. Turn half way through cooking with tongs.
6. Drain eggplant on paper towel, then transfer to serving dish. Transfer honey to serving dish.
7. Serve hot.

Deer Jerky

Prep Time: 10 minutes*
Dehydrating Time: 4 - 8 hours
Servings: 4

INGREDIENTS

4 oz (1/4 lb) grass-fed beef

2 tablespoons coconut aminos (or liquid aminos or tamari)

2 tablespoons lemon juice (or apple cider vinegar or coconut vinegar)

1 teaspoon raw honey (or agave or date butter)

1/2 teaspoon onion powder

1/2 teaspoon garlic powder

1 teaspoon Hungarian hot paprika (or paprika)

1 teaspoon ground black pepper

2 teaspoons Celtic sea salt

INSTRUCTIONS

1. Prepare two parchment sheets. Lay one on cutting board.
2. Slice venison into 1/4 inch strips and lay in single layer on parchment. Pound with tenderizing side of kitchen mallet. Cover venison with second parchment sheet, then pound with flat side of tenderizing mallet to 1/8 inch thickness.
3. *Place venison strips in medium mixing bowl or shallow dish. Add coconut aminos, lemon juice, honey, salt and spices. Mix well to coat. Cover and place in refrigerator for 8 hours, or overnight.

4. Remove meat from refrigerator and lay in single layer on dehydrator trays. Place in dehydrator and dehydrate at 120 degrees F for 4 - 8 hours.
5. After 4 hours dehydrating time, remove trays from dehydrator and test jerky by bending. If it cracks, remove and serve immediately. Or store in airtight container.
6. If still flexible, place back in dehydrator and continue dehydrating up to 4 hours, or until desired texture is achieved.

Primal Cocoa Zucchini Muffin

Prep Time: 10 minutes

Cook Time: 15 minutes

Servings: 12

INGREDIENTS

1 1/2 cups almond flour

2 cage-free eggs

1 small zucchini (about 1 cup grated)

1/2 cup unsweetened applesauce

1/4 cup date butter (or agave or raw honey)

1/4 cup coconut oil (or cacao or coconut butter, melted)

1/4 cup cocoa powder

2 tablespoons ground chia seed (or flax meal)

1 teaspoon baking soda

1 teaspoon baking powder

1 teaspoon vanilla

1 teaspoon ground cinnamon

1 teaspoon ground black pepper

1/2 teaspoon Celtic sea salt

1/4 cup cocoa nibs or chocolate chips (optional)

INSTRUCTIONS

1. Preheat oven to 350 degrees F. Line muffin pan with paper liners or lightly coat with coconut oil.

2. Add eggs, oil or melted butter, applesauce and date butter to food processor or high-speed blender. Process until thick, light mixture forms, about 1 - 2 minutes.
3. Sift almond flour, cocoa powder, chia or flax meal, baking soda and powder, salt and spices into processor. Process to combine, about 1 minute.
4. Grate zucchini and stir in with cocoa nibs or chocolate chips (optional).
5. Use scoop or tablespoon to pour batter into prepared muffin pan. Bake for about 15 - 20 minutes, until toothpick inserted into center comes out clean.
6. Remove from oven and let cool about 5 minutes.
7. Serve warm. Or let cool completely and serve room temperature.

Olive Tapenade

Prep Time: 15 minutes

Servings: 2

INGREDIENTS

1 1/2 cups any combination pitted olives (Kalamata, Spanish, black, pimento, etc.)

2 tablespoons capers

2 anchovy fillets

1 garlic clove

2 fresh basil leaves

1/2 lemon

2 tablespoons coconut oil

INSTRUCTIONS

1. Peel garlic and add to food processor or high-speed blender. Process until finely ground.
2. Rinse and drain olives, capers and anchovy fillets. Add to processor with basil, oil and squeeze of 1/2 lemon. Process until finely chopped or coarsely ground, about 1 - 2 minutes.
3. Transfer to serving dish and serve immediately.

Gingerbread Cookies

Prep Time: 5 minutes

Cook Time: 15 minutes

Servings: 12

INGREDIENTS

1 cup almond flour

2 cage-free eggs

1/2 cup dried pitted dates

1/4 cup raw honey (or dark agave)

1/4 cup coconut oil (or cacao butter, melted)

1/2 teaspoon baking soda

1/2 teaspoon baking powder

2 teaspoons ground ginger

1 teaspoon ground cinnamon

1 teaspoon vanilla

1/2 teaspoon ground cloves

1/2 teaspoon ground black pepper

1/4 teaspoon Celtic sea salt

Natural sarsaparilla or root beer beverage, or nut milk (optional)

INSTRUCTIONS

1. Preheat oven to 350 degrees F. Line sheet pan with parchment or baking mat.

2. Add dates, honey or agave and eggs to food processor or high-speed blender. Process until thick smooth mixture forms, about 2 minutes.
3. Add almond flour, oil or butter, baking soda and powder, salt and spices to processor. Process until thick mixture comes together, about 1 minute. Add sarsaparilla, root beer or nut milk to thin as necessary. Batter should resemble thick cookie dough.
4. From rounds and place on prepares sheet pan. Flatten into disks.
5. Bake 10 - 15 minutes, until browned around edges and cooked through, but still soft.
6. Remove from oven and let cool at about 10 minutes.
7. Transfer to serving dish and serve warm. Or cool completely and serve room temperature.

Spicy Chicken Wraps

Prep time: 5 minutes

Cook time: 3 minutes

INGREDIENTS

4 slices of chicken deli meat

1 tbsp olive oil

1 small onion

1 red bell pepper

1 avocado

¼ tsp garlic powder

INSTRUCTIONS

1. Remove the nut from the avocado and mash it into a paste. Chop the pepper and onion into small pieces.
2. Combine the garlic powder, pepper and onion in the bowl with the avocado and mix well.
3. Add the olive oil in a pan over low heat and heat the chicken mildly, turning frequently, for 3 minutes.
4. Remove the chicken from heat and place ¼ of the avocado/pepper/onion mixture onto each piece.
5. Wrap the chicken up into tubes and serve.

Tahini with Fruit Topping

Prep time: 4 minutes

INGREDIENTS

1 large celery stalk

¼ cup tahini

2 tsp cinnamon

½ cup blueberries

½ cup strawberries

INSTRUCTIONS

1. In a small bowl, mix the cinnamon into the tahini. Wash the celery stalk and dry the concave inside. Chop the strawberries.
2. Spread the tahini mixture throughout the concave inside.
3. Stick the fruit into the tahini side by side alternating blueberry/strawberry.
4. Serve.

Sugar Free Baked Apples

Prep time: 10 minutes

Cook time: 20-25 minutes

Servings: 2

INGREDIENTS

3 apples

¼ cup raisins

¼ cup chopped almonds (or walnuts)

½ cup water

1 tbsp lemon juice

½ tsp cinnamon

¼ tsp ginger

raw, unfiltered honey

INSTRUCTIONS

1. Preheat oven to 350 degrees.
2. Slice and core apples. Place in an 8x8 baking pan. Pour water and lemon juice over the apples and let sit in baking dish. Sprinkle raisins, almonds/walnuts, ginger and cinnamon over the top. Cover with tin foil and bake for 20-25 minutes or until apple is tender.
3. Remove from oven and serve in a bowl with honey drizzled over the top.

Ginger Mango Sherbet

Prep Time: 5* minutes

Cook Time: 15 minutes

Servings: 4

INGREDIENTS

1 cup almond milk

1 cup coconut milk

2 ripe mangos

2 oz fresh ginger juice (about 8 inch bunch ginger root)

Juice of lime half

Zest of lime half

1 teaspoon vanilla

Bunch fresh mint

INSTRUCTIONS

1. *Freeze ice cream maker canister overnight before to make sure it is cold enough.
2. Add whole peeled ginger root to food processor. Or juice ginger and add to medium mixing bowl. Add mint leaves.
3. Slice, pit and peel mangos. Add to food processor or bullet blender with almond milk. Blend or process until smooth, then strain into medium mixing bowl.
4. Add coconut milk, juice and zest of half a lime, and vanilla. Mix well with whisk or hand mixer.

5. Turn on ice cream maker first, then carefully pour in mango mixture as ice cream maker paddle rotates.
6. Freeze for about 15 - 20 minutes. Then transfer frozen custard to serving dishes.
7. Serve immediately.

Basic Banana Bread

Prep Time: 5 minutes

Cook Time: 40 minutes

Servings: 8

INGREDIENTS

1 cup almond flour

1/4 cup coconut flour

2 overripe bananas

2 cage-free eggs

1/4 cup agave nectar (or stevia)

1/4 cup unsweetened applesauce

1 tablespoon baking powder

2 teaspoons ground cinnamon

1/2 teaspoon ground nutmeg

1 teaspoon vanilla

1/2 teaspoon Celtic sea salt

INSTRUCTIONS

1. Preheat oven to 350 degrees F. Coat small or medium loaf pan with coconut oil.
2. Peel bananas and add to medium mixing bowl. Beat with hand mixer or whisk. Add eggs, applesauce, and sweetener. Beat well, about 1 - 2 minutes.
3. In separate bowl, blend flours, baking powder, salt and spices. Pour banana mixture into flour mixture and stir to combine.

4. Pour batter into prepared loaf pan and bake for 30 - 40 minutes, or until browned and firm in the center.
5. Remove from oven and set aside to cool.
6. Slice and serve warm. Or allow to cool completely and serve room temperature.

Made in the USA
Columbia, SC
06 May 2020